Living with Scleroderma

Living with Scleroderma

Introduction

This is my personal experience living with the diagnosis of Scleroderma starting from age twenty five. I was diagnosed with what they call Limited Scleroderma or formerly known as CREST.

I decided to write this book to help others cope with the daily challenges of this horrific disease where no cure is in sight.

This book is written from a patients point of view, mine!

I would like to remind you that this is how I'm living with Scleroderma. I'm not recommending you try my coping skills, nor that you agree with how I continue to survive this dreadful disease for thirty years. I'm merely sharing with you, how I'm winning this daily fight as a patient, wife, mother and author.

Since only the symptoms can be addressed with this diagnosis. I kept a journal to keep track of how it effected my body and inner peace. Do you have hope? Are you scared? Are your fingers tight? Are you feeling lost? Do you feel embarrassed? Does your Doctor really know what to do? Am I going to die? I know there are many questions you're asking yourself.

The prognosis for CREST is, eleven years after onset comes death. So, find a coping mechanism, because you're not dying, at least not today.

For me, I say... be filled with hope through what ever comes your way. It's a hard ride, but I must confess, each challenge led me elsewhere, and that pushed me evolve. I gained knowledge and strength.

Books Written By:Sharon Marie Bence

- Twisted Testimonials

- Thought I Knew The Plan

- Living with Scleroderma

- Twisted Testimonials #2 (Coming Soon)

Chapter One

Remembering that year, was so crystal clear...Twenty five, pregnant, and in the middle of a divorce. If that wasn't enough stress for one person, I don't know what is.

On this particular Wednesday I was on my way to a doctors appointment. I noticed a hard lump growing on my forearm. It wasn't painful, just bothersome.

Pulling open the heavy glass door, I walked over to the reception desk to sign in.

"Ms. Bence." Called the blonde wearing my favorite color scrubs. Politely she began asking about my past medical history for the doctor. Then the doctor came in just as I began reading an article about landscaping.

"Good afternoon. How can I help you today?" I showed him my forearm. He asked me a ton of questions while examining my arms and legs.

"I think you might have an autoimmune disease. Its called Scleroderma. Do you know what that is?" Shaking my head no, he proceeded.

"I won't know for sure until I take blood tests. Here's a pamphlet. You can read up on it, and see me in two weeks."

Thanking him, I grabbed the information and headed to the dressing room to change.

Before I could go home, I needed to go to the grocery store.

Home at last, I put the food away. Taking a breather, I sat down to read the paper about the disease. The pamphlet had minimal information. So, I looked it up on the web.

As I read the screen, it spoke about the symptoms, and that it was a rare disease. After reading that sentence, I became more inquisitive, so I searched for all information I could find. I was so surprised when I read the prognosis, my mouth dropped open. The prognosis was DEATH. After I read it, I threw the pamphlet in the trash, and said "Lord, you take this." and I gave it to God.

What does that mean, give it to God? It's important for you understand this. It's the foundation of how I handled the confirmation of having Scleroderma and all of life's major issues.

For me, it means letting go of situations I can't control. It means not worrying about the diagnosis, or anything else. Knowing deep in your heart that Jesus healed you two thousand years ago when he hung on the cross. My healing is of supernatural favor. I'm under his saving grace.

I know its easier said than done. But, I also know that constant stress, worry and pain will accelerate this disease. Learning how to deal with stress and pain on a daily basis is so important.

It's also beneficial to distance people or issues causing you stress. Peace, has to become your ultimate goal while learning various methods to calm the pain and progression of this horrible disease.

We each have to make a choice. Are you going to give up and let the disease take you, or are you going to be a fighter?

Chapter Two

A few years later I noticed my hands and feet were always cold. It didn't matter if it was summer or winter. It didn't matter if I wore gloves or not. My circulation was poor and the winters up north were taking a toll on my body. Below zero temperatures and blowing freezing winds became a very big problem for me. My hands and feet would turn blue, go numb and ache terribly.

My regular physician referred me to a Rhumatologist, who informed me it was Reynauds Syndrome. This was the second symptom. The calcinosis that was growing on my forearm was the first sign.

After going through many stressful life changes, my symptoms began to increase intensely. Calcinosis began growing on my kneecaps, the tips of my fingers and my ears.

Sometimes a hot bath with Epsom salt helped. I soon found out that I had to become my own surgeon. I began picking, cutting or tweezing the calcium out of my skin myself to relieve the constant pain and pressure of the calcinosis.

I must admit the extraction was very painful and at times I couldn't believe the size and sharpness of the pieces. Some were half the size as my kneecap. Each day a little at a time some would surface to the top layers of my skin. I would remove it, clean it well and cover it with a band aid. It left me with many scars but the relief of having it out of my body was worth it.

Remember, if you do try to remove pieces yourself, make sure you have a sterile tool. Infection is the last thing you want to bring upon yourself.

For me, that's one of the most frustrating issues as a patient. Having this foreign growth, pressing on your nerves and no help available except surgery. I was told that even if you get it removed surgically, it grows back. I'm proof it does. I think you would agree with me, this disease is No Fun!

The doctor's I seen couldn't find any medications to increase my circulation nor prevent the growth of calcium. I took many medications to try to address the symptoms but, none stopped the calcium from growing and my extremities were getting worse.

I wasn't much on taking medication. I hated to take pills. I added homeopathic practices into my regime to reach past the prescriptions. But it didn't work. I changed my diet by adding more foods for the brain and immune system, such as blueberries, kale, avocado and walnuts. I then started smoking medical marijuana for my pain.

That same year, my finger tip became infected by an ulcer formed by the calcium under my nail bed. They put me on a high dose of antibiotics and steroids. I couldn't believe my own finger tip was disappearing before my very eyes. It looked as though it was being eaten away, and it felt like it too! It was extremely hard to continue with my daily tasks such as going to work, taking care of my child, driving and cooking.

I had to become conscious of NOT using my finger when I had to do a task. I became quickly aware each time I accidentally hit it or grabbed something wrong. The pain would literally double me over.

This was the week I had a doctor appointment to check my fingertip. I'd been nursing it for sixty days while on antibiotics.

"Sharon, I'm afraid your finger isn't healing and it's starting to turn gangrene."

My facial expression was confused. What does that mean I thought?

Gangrene: Localized death and decomposition of body tissue, resulting from either obstructed circulation or bacterial infection. {Google Definition}

He told me he was referring me to a hand surgeon for surgery. I begged and pleaded with him not to have it amputated. I reassured him over and over that I could care for it, and it would heal. But, he wouldn't hear of it because of the infection. After he told me it could spread through my body, I knew it was completely necessary, and I reluctantly agreed.

It was an out patient procedure, not a complicated surgery. I was happy with the surgeons outcome. My finger didn't take very long to heal. Before I knew it, I was back to work. The type of work I did at the time required a lot of typing. I learned how to adapt to an amputated tip and most people never even realized it was removed.

I thank God it didn't interfere with my ability to continue life routines at work and at home. I didn't let it effect my self worth. I got depressed about it, from time to time.

But, we're only human. I patiently waited and let it heal. I also adapted to how I used my right hand and then I gave it to God.

Both Doctors told me the cold climate was not good for my poor circulation. I had thought about moving for years. Somewhere sunnier and some where warmer. Maybe this year I should considerate it, I thought.

Chapter Three

Five Years Later...

Still not being unable to function well in the winter, I decided to move out of the state to a warmer climate. After 5 years, still there were no medications that worked to help with my circulation or calcinosis.

I finally found a new Rheumatologest. She was from Romania and she had the best bedside manner. She truly was one of those doctors that took the time to listen and cared what was going on.

I remember one time, I was sitting in her office with tears rolling down my cheeks. She gave me a hug and assured me everything would be alright. Since I had to see her every three months, she was well informed of my condition.

The next symptoms showed up about a year later, acid reflux and the tiny red dots that were popping up on my face, hands and mouth. They called this symptom, Talangiectasia. I started eating antacids like candy until my doctor put me on Prilosec. I ignored the tiny red dots, they didn't bother me. Each time I looked in the mirror, my face was changing. I wasn't a vain person. I knew my beauty was within, so I gave it to God.

On this particular day she took a chance and fought with the insurance to put me on Sidenafil (Viagra) for my circulation. She got some backlash from the insurance but, she wasn't going to give up. That was the first, and only medication that worked to increase my blood flow, and I still take it today thirty years later. Now that she found a medication that helped my circulation, she informed me that there were no good options for the calcinosis. I must admit, the warmer climate did help with my circulation.

For several years I just had minor issues that I could contain. Until my next test, a bone scan. That test came back, and I was diagnosed with Osteoporosis.

She immediately put me on Prolia shots once a year. After the first year, she did a bone scan to see if the Prolia was working.
The bone density test confirmed it was indeed, growing new bone.

I was amazed and thought, what a miracle. Yes, I still had to deal with the calcinosis but it was manageable at that time. I was determined that it wasn't going to stop me.

There were times I felt fatigued, but I pushed myself when I needed, and rested when my body told me to. I found out that it was very important to listen to what my body was trying to tell me and to follow it's cue. I began to command my body to repair itself routinely.

My faith in God took me to a deeper spiritual level. I was finding I was enjoying life. I found most of my serenity in nature. I truly love flowers with a passion, and the smell of fresh cut grass is a heavenly fragrance to me.

It was my time to enjoy nature in the warm sun. Strangely enough, it seemed that when I did what I enjoyed, the pain of my fingers would disappear. I could work for hours and not think about the disease. It's as if my soul was joyfully working in the dirt, and my human hands were not an issue.

"I am healed through Jesus stripes." I would say over and over. After, I would order my cells to stop fighting and aline. Meditation and yoga were helpful too. As long as I kept moving and kept believing, all was well. I continued to take my medication and take care of my body, mind and spirit.

For years there were no major issues, until I was having trouble swallowing. Another test was in order. This one was rather cool. I could see on the monitor each time I swallowed. What they found was a delay in the swallowing process. When I ate, food didn't automatically go directly down my esophagus. I had to be conscious of this while I ate. I learned to eat smaller meals, smaller bites and to slow down my pace.

I was diagnosed with Barrett disease and had my esophagus burned to remove the black growth that covered the skin. This is when the acid splashes up into the esophagus. It was two weeks before I could eat. That hurt a lot!

Chapter Four

At this point in time I had lived with Scleroderma for fifteen years.
It was a normal Wednesday and I was at the doctor thinking about what I needed to tell her.

At work I was having great difficulty typing and carrying files. It was hard to even remove the files from the filing cabinet. My coworkers were coming in over the weekend to catch up. My boss asked if I could help. I sat in front of her, trying not to cry as I began my explanation.

"Physically I don't feel I could help."
She listened as I explained my disease. She looked at my hands and seen the deformity from the calcinosis, and she sympathized.

"Why didn't you tell me sooner you were hurting so bad?"
I explained to her how I try my best not to complain or even acknowledge the disease

because it gives the disease power over me. She gave me a hug, and told me to keep her updated on what the doctor says, as I headed to see her.

"Hello dear. How are you feeling today?" I began to cry.
She knew that I was a woman who kept a positive attitude and wondered what I was so upset about. I showed her my index finger with the ulcer on it.

"Oh my, that looks so painful Sharon. I think it's time to stop working dear and file for disability."

I was in shock. I didn't even know what disability was. She explained it to me while handing me a Kleenex.

"I think you'll be better off not having to try and work with the ulcer and the pain in your hands. Your diagnosis does qualify you, and I will make sure you get it." She checked the ulcer, it wasn't infected yet. It looked as though a wild animal had been forcefully gnawing on my finger for months. An open wound, different levels of the skin missing and tiny pieces of calcium trying to make it's way out.

I left her office feeling defeated by the disease. I cried all the way to my car as I mulled over in my mind the next step I had to take.

"What would I do without work? Who would I be? What about my bills?" In that very instant, I drove by a statue of Jesus. He reminded me that he had my back. So, I took a deep breath and once again, I gave it to God.

When I arrived home I went directly to my laptop and filed for disability on the website. It was a very lengthy process that required a lot of detailed information. I was determined to get it finished and filed that day. Using my fourth fingers to peck out the answers, I felt like my hands were burning like fire afterwards. This proved to me that although I was scared, I needed to listen to the doctor and trust that it all would work out.

After I sent in the form I pondered again, who will I be without my job? Society puts so much focus on what we do for a living. It becomes our identity. The first thing someone asks you when you're getting to know them is,

"What do you do for a living?" What would I say? Who am I? Disabled didn't sound like a worthy title. After working for twenty five years. I believe at that very moment, my old life style was at an end, and a new journey was about to begin.

It took me years reprogramming my thinking. I needed to learn how not to conform to society's rules. I had to keep my focus on God's plan. Don't fall into society's tricks.

You are not just a body, or what you do for a living. You are spirit with a mission and capable of all things through Jesus Christ.

Chapter Five

My boss put me on light duty while my ulcer was wrapped and well cushioned. I shared with my boss my doctors advice to file for disability. She asked me to keep her informed.

When I returned home I took off the wrap and gave it some air. I was given Silver Sulfadiazine to put on my ulcer two times a day. For me, that cream was a life saver. It's what they use on burn patients. It was so soothing on the wound that I applied it more than prescribed. I was given pain medication as well. My sleep became disturbed and my appetite was not up to par. It was getting harder to wake up on time for work.

Deciding to walk down the street to check the mail, the box was stuffed full. Shuffling through all the junk as I walked home, I noticed a letter from Social Security. To my horrible dismay, I was denied. My heart dropped into my stomach. Thinking, what now?

The very next day I called the Social Security office to make an appointment for them to help me fill out the form. At this point I could no longer peck at the keys to type. The lady was very courteous and helpful. I informed my boss when my next appointment was scheduled.

I was eager to get the form filed. Overhearing two men talking about how almost everyone gets turned down the first time you file, gave me some hope.

The following day my boss told me that she had to hire someone else for my position. She was sweet and understanding. She didn't want to see me go, but since I could not do my job, she was doing both our jobs and needed help.

The very next day I filed for SSI to get me by financially. I was accepted and assured that I had money coming in for the bills. I left my job for the unknown. It was scary. I felt like I wasn't worthy anymore. Who was I? A question that kept haunting my mind. I didn't know. I didn't have any idea. I could tell people my past, but my present was unknown.

About six months later I received a letter from Social Security. I was fearful to open it. I was so afraid they'd turned me down again. SSI was temporary. I was receiving food stamps as well. I was very grateful for the state programs I qualified for. But, at the same time I felt down on myself for having to use the programs because I always had pride in supporting myself.

Pushing aside the fear, I took a deep breath and opened the letter slowly. Reading, filled with anxiety, I reached the area where it said, "You Qualify." A huge smile appeared as tears of happiness streamed down my face. I was so grateful! I thanked God for his help. I could now rest knowing my bills would be paid.

Chapter Six

Disability Approved

For a good month my body enjoyed sleeping in until I woke up naturally, no alarm. My day was filled with rest, prayer and watching television. I began reading the bible online. I was becoming closer to Jesus and chatting with him about my fears regularly.

In a month my finger ulcer was healed. I didn't have the same mobilization I once had. The nail bed was completely gone and along with my nail falling off my finger it became contorted with little to no dexterity. It looked as though a chainsaw accidentally nicked it.

At times, I felt like I could just scream due to the pain and there were times I did. There were also times I've cried myself to sleep.

Being on disability gave me free time that I never had before. Finding out it was great for my body, but not so much for my mind. I began feeling lonely. Depression fell upon me too and I wasn't sure where to take my life. What would I do with my time? How would I live on a limited income? I wondered.

It was very difficult adjusting to not being on a working schedule, when you have been all of your life. When I had to fill out a form, and it asks for your occupation, I would put disabled. Each time I did, I felt lost, like I was grieving the loss of my identity. I asked God, "What should I do now Lord?"

Having one finger amputated, and calcium consuming my body. I was beside myself. I could always tell where the calcinosis was. Not usually the depth but, when they were surfacing to the top. Having The pieces in the first and second layer of skin were easy to detect. Those deeper, were always a waiting game to see if they would surface. The wait of not knowing if the wound would heal, or turn gangrene is a horror I live with still today.

I would do the best I could to keep the wounds clean. I prayed and repeated in my mind, I am healed by his stripes. I would also repeat, my cells are coming together to make my immune system stronger. I thanked Jesus for my healing routinely. Especially before bedtime when I knew I was in for a long nights fight to find comfort.

It was imperative that I believed I was healed no matter what I seen or felt. My goal has been to train my brain to believe what my heart did. I was healed.

I know your thinking, how can you believe your healed when your symptoms are everywhere? I agree it's a hard concept to understand. But, I knew that choosing to have my faith scared and becoming depressed wouldn't give me a fighting chance for survival. My mom always said, "You can lay down and die or you can fight."

I am a fighter and you have to be too!

Chapter Seven

A few years later, due to a family situation, I found myself having to move back to the cold northern air in Kansas. I rented my house, packed my belongings and hit the road.

This move was a life changing experience. I had so much change and stress in that one year that it left my immune system striped. I lost a 14 year relationship and my daughter was soon to give birth to her first child. It was just her and I on this journey.

The summer months were comfortable but the chill in the fall air made my hands turn white, go numb then turn blue. This concerned me so I told my doctor. Every three months I continued to see my Rhumatologist. At this time in my life, there still was no cure to stop the calcinosis from growing or preventing the calcium from turning into ulcers.

I had often wondered if lazer surgery

would be able to break up or dissolve the calcinosis. It was not something anyone had ever tried. Sidnifil was 99% effective in the warm climate. It really helped me a lot. However, in below zero temperatures it did not stop the symptom of Reynauds.

My daughter gave birth to a beautiful baby girl. I got to cut the cord. It was the most amazing experience I ever had in my life besides giving birth to my own. From that minute when I became a grandma, I had a new purpose. Her birth brought me joy and happiness.

That winter was not good to me. My feet were also turning blue and a piece of calcium in my third and fourth toe on my right foot was forming an ulcer. Back and forth in the freezing cold and snow to see my Rhumatologist for months. My toes were unable to be saved. They became infected and turned gangrene.

Since I had gone through this with my finger, I knew I was heading into long suffering.

The doctor scheduled me to have my toes amputated. I decided to return south. Back to my home rather than have the surgery there.

The next step was to call my Realtor and explain how desperately I needed to come home and asked her to speak to the renters. To my surprise, they needed to move as well. The timing was perfect. That was God.

Chapter Eight

The surgery was performed with my faith in tact. I was ready. They were to remove a few toes. However, the infection had gone further than they had anticipated. To my horror, I was left with only half of my foot. I was in the hospital for a week.

Such pain shot through the tightly wrapped bandages. I had not seen my foot, nor was this pain, something I ever felt. It was like having a knife stabbed in my foot with someone turning it deeper into my skin. I was irritable and angry.

When the surgeon came to speak to me I asked him when I could see the wound and I shared with him my pain level.

"That's normal pain for an amputation. You see, we had to cut off more than I had anticipated. The infection from the toes traveled up to mid foot. We also removed the calcinosis on the heel of your foot. It was six inches deep, and at your request we removed the huge piece on your forearm."

His orders were written for wound care twice a week at home and 3 times a week with the wound doctor. I was discharged with a walker and a hand shake. I left the hospital in complete anger and shock.

The next day when I awoke, I stood up out of the bed as normal, but fell flat on my face. My brain did not recognize that my foot was amputated. Very confused, I sat on the floor asking myself, "Why did I just fall?" In the distance I seen my walker at the end of my bed.

To me, it felt like the surgery was a nightmare I couldn't wake up from. However, seeing the walker proved to me it was indeed reality.

Frustrated, I and carefully crawled to the walker being aware not to loosen the bandages. While using the bed as a brace, pulling with all my upper arm strength, I got up. Bracing, trying to get my balance steady, I began to take my first step, and I fell again! You see, I understood cognitively that I had only half a foot but again, my brain denied it.

Sitting on the floor puzzled, weeping, frustrated and in pain. I wiped my tears, thought strategically about how to get up with one working leg. This time with a plan, pulling myself up, then bracing myself with my good leg, I sat at the end of the bed and rested before trying to walk again.

Chapter Nine

My family stayed the first couple days to help me prepare meals and assist me In and out of the tub. This particular Monday was the day the nurse would come to clean my wound. Today was the day I would finally get to see my foot for the first time. I was anxious and in severe pain as I hopped around the house on one foot getting myself presentable. I was exhausted after just doing that little bit of moving.

The doorbell rung just as I had finished getting ready. My daughter opened the door.

"Hi Sharon. I'm Judy and I'll be your nurse today. How did your surgery go?"

"I think it went well. I haven't seen what it looks like yet.

"That's good. I'll be unwrapping it today,

cleaning and taking notes on the progress of healing. I see here that you will be attending wound care three times a week"

Focused, she removed a folder filled with paperwork that I needed to sign before we began. Politely she took my blood pressure and temperature. She made a notation, then explained what I was signing and why.

She had a sunny disposition and a soft caring voice that made me smile and feel at ease. "Let me know if you start to feel any pain and I'll stop. What would you say your level of pain is right now?"

"I'd say about a 5. I'm scared to see it." I admitted in fear.

Starting to unravel the gauze slowly one layer at a time we chatted nonchalantly. Lifting my foot for stabilization, sent me into outer space, I jumped right out off the chair. The nerves at the bottom of my foot felt like she was stabbing me with a butcher knife and turning it counter clockwise! I could feel my teeth clinch as she asked, "Are you alright?"

Nodding my head yes, she proceeded. On the last piece of gauze that was pushed into the wound, I closed my eyes as she pulled with a forceful tug.

"Oh my God that hurts! Ow, Ow, Ow! Can you pour some saline solution to loosen the gauze." I could feel the dried blood and wound discharge tearing off the edges of the stump. With my eyes still closed she cleaned the wound and very gently pulled out the remaining gauze.

"Ouch, that hurts!"

"I'm sorry Sharon, but I got it. Are you ready to open your eyes and take a look?"

My pain level that was a five, was now a ten. Tears were involuntary dripping. I really didn't want to open my eyes. I didn't want this to be my reality. I wanted to go back to work and be free of such excruciating pain. This must be a bad dream, I thought in a state of panic as I uncovered my eyes.

Both my hands instantly cupped my mouth as I let out a deep gasp of shock. Tears fell rapidly with dismay and loss. I cant tell you, what I thought I'd see, but what I saw, I was not prepared to see.

My foot was cut all the way back past my arch. The wound was black, wide and deep. Just being exposed to the air alone was pure pain. Unable to get over the immediate shock, Judy gave me a hug and assured me that she'd seen worse and that It would be okay.

I thanked her for her support, then she left. I was mortified. Everything was gone. The sight made me nauseated.
I knew this was the beginning of some very difficult changes.

Chapter Ten

Scleroderma like most diseases are cruel. If you let it, it can steal your worth. The seconds of each day putting up with constant pain and constant scarring can zap your energy both mentally and physically. Depression and a loss of hope can set in when you're told the same thing over and over again... there is no cure, I'm sorry.

If you are one that worries a lot, don't! It will increase your stress. In turn, making the body unbalanced and increasing symptoms of calcinosis can result in a lower immune system.

Unfortunately, this disease never went into remission. Did you notice, I chose the word disease verses, my disease. That's because in my mind, I Do Not Claim It. What is she talking about you're probably wondering? Remember how I mentioned in the beginning of the book that having faith in Jesus, that unshakable kind of faith, that put your foot down kind of faith.

Well, my faith in him is just that! I am not moved by what I see on my body long term. I thank him every day for opening up my eyes. I fully believe he gets me through every single day. I believe he went to heaven and back for us. I believe that I am healed from any one or thing that wants to bring me ill will.
I believe when he was gasping for air in his last breath he spoke.

"Its finished."
It was finished, and I was healed. All I had to do was believe it. Claim it. Thank him for his healing hand and the plans he has for my future.

That's the hard part. Staying steadfast in his words of promise. But, how can one do that when I look at myself in the mirror and I see the scars mixed with current calcium outbreaks on my chin, cheek and forehead.

I look down and see two amputated fingers and three deformed from the calcium and now my foot.

How can I stay positive, how can I get through? So much pain and I'm on my own.

My struggles were in many forms from as little as holding a glass to bathing and cooking.

My first day driving with my left foot

instead of right took some practice. But over time it became second nature. Riding in an electric grocery cart became the norm and I hated it! Just like when my handicap placard came in the mail. I felt was a sinking feeling in my gut hearing those words officially
   "Disabled."
 This disease throws you a lot of different punches. It hits your self worth, your physical abilities and health as well as your mental health. You must become a warrior and remain open minded for what works for you.

Chapter Eleven

My first wound care appointment was today. I was a little nervous not knowing what I would encounter. I made it driving by myself safely. In order to do that, I took off my right shoe so it wasn't in the way. I drove with it tucked under my left leg. Then I utilized my left foot to operate the pedals.

The nurse put me in a very cold room painted baby blue. The dividing curtain hung from the ceiling was blue too with a sea shell design. Everyone was quite polite and helpful.

I didn't take very long before the nurse came in to ask be some questions about the amputation. She gently unwrapped the lawyers of bandages and gauze. The feeling of my foot being free was painful when the air hit it. I became very guarded over my wound. She took my vital signs. But before she left, I asked her for a blanket. I was freezing and my feet were starting to turn blue. I knew this symptom wasn't good. The nurse obliged and the next nurse walked in with the doctor. Holding my foot tight, protecting it with both hands I could feel my foot begin throbbing. A painful tingling sensation that turned into a burning knife stabbing pain along the open wound.

The Doctor looked at the nurses notes and asked me a few questions. "I've treated open wounds like this before. I'm sure in about three months of therapy you should be healed. Do you see this part? It's all black dead skin and we want a pretty pink flesh to grow back."

Smiling, I asked "How do we get the pretty pink tissue?"

"Good question. Do you see these instruments? As she disrobed the green cloth that covered the sterile tools. I glanced over and knew each one. I could see tweezers, mirror, scissors, gauze and a silver pick. I shook my head yes.

"The tweezers and pick is what I'll be using to remove the dead skin so new skin will replace it. So, tell me when you're ready and we'll get started."

No better time than now, I thought. "I'm ready." Still holding my foot stable, I let go reluctantly. Turning my attention towards the pretty blue curtain I ignored what was about to happen to my foot. The doctor took her first pull at the dead skin, I jumped to the ceiling.

All my nerve's were exposed and I was livid.

"My dear God, that hurts!" Seeing her go for another tug, I closed my eyes and waited for the pain. Biting my lip I tested my endurance and tolerance.

She had jerked many pieces of dead skin, as I focused on the colorful curtain. Cringing and with tears slowly dripping from my eyes, I asked "Can I take a break? I'm really hurting!" Looking at the clock in surprise, "Wow, I've been working for almost an hour. That went by fast, don't you think?" She smiled.

"Not fast enough."

"Well, we will be seeing you three times a week Sharon. Make your appointment at the desk when you leave. You did very good for your first time. Have a good day."

The nurse came in to clean and re wrap my amputation. She was gentle and apologized for hurting me. Still sniffling, she said "It will get easier with time. You're gonna be okay. I think we should get you some crutches and take that walker away. Who gave that to you anyway?"

"The hospital after surgery."

"I bet that's hard hop, get your balance and than hop again. I think you'll find the crutches much easier. I'll be right back."
She came back quickly with a pair of crutches. Fitting them to my size, she nodded her head in

approval. "Now, that's what I'm talking about! I bet that feels ten times better."

Putting them under my arms and tucking my right leg behind me sure was a lot better than using the walker. I thanked her, and she gave me a hug." You have a nice rest of your day ma'am"

As I got in the elevator I realized that nurse was special. She gave me hope and the hug, I needed so desperately. I was so happy to get rid of that walker, it was the highlight of my day. Driving, I noticed a statue of Jesus on the right on Ocean Boulevard. Passing by I thanked him for being with me during this extremely difficult situation. Heading home with a smile, it felt good to be more mobile.

Chapter Twelve

Not having an appetite and my pain deliriously high, I decided to take a nap. Hopping down the long hallway, leaning my crutches against the wall, I took one Oxycontin and fell asleep. I was still having difficulty sleeping since the surgery. Sometimes just the bed sheet touching my wound would make me want to scream and that's with the wound wrapped, which it constantly was except when the dressing was changed. Often I couldn't find a comfortable position.

I'd sleep at the head of the bed, the bottom of the bed and sideways. Sideways seemed preferable because my feet weren't touching anything, just hanging off the bed. Another reason why I wasn't sleeping was because the phantom pains would shoot right through me like fire. Sometimes it felt like my toes were cramping like a charlie horse.

Logically, I knew they were gone, yet I

rubbed my foot to stop the spasms. At best I guess you could say I was becoming an insomniac.

Five hours later I opened my eyes in the dark. I was a confused so I took a minute to sit up and orient myself. Standing up to reach for my crutches, I fell. The only thing I hurt was my pride, I was okay. Crawling on the ground to get my crutches I learned not to set them so far away from the bed. Turning on the lights in the living room I noticed it was nine thirty PM. I felt somewhat hungry so I fixed myself a sandwich and poured an ice tea and watched the news. At this particular time, the in-home nurse was canceled.

The wound clinic would change the wrappings during the week. I would be responsible for two days on the weekend. It still turned my stomach to look at the wound especially being able to see the exposed bone. The doctor only got a tiny corner of dead skin debrided last visit. This is going to take forever I thought

Where I once had toes, remained a half of foot. This wound was deep and black everywhere. The process was so intense! "I think I'll ask tomorrow if they have some sort of numbing cream to put on before she starts ripping off my skin.

After watching the news, I wrapped my

foot with a plastic bag, took a shower and went to my bed. Tomorrow was another early wound therapy day. I sat on the edge of my bed leaning the crutches close by and lit a medical marijuana cigarette. I rolled over the day in my mind. I was exhausted and hoped I could sleep a full eight hours.

Chapter Thirteen

Hitting the snooze button repeatedly, the fifth time, I reluctantly got up. Seeing the crutches in my peripheral vision I grabbed them."That makes life a little better" I murmured. Slowly hopping to the kitchen, getting my coffee ready, I grabbed my keys and got on the road.

It was a beautiful summer day and I loved the drive that took me over the bay into the city. The traffic was light was my exit.

"Good morning Jesus." I said after I drove past his statue on my way.

Debating in my mind how to accomplish taking my coffee in with me while hopping into the waiting room without spilling it was a big dilemma. It seemed like every day there was a new challenge I had to solve or adapt to.

Life was no longer the same, and never

would be. Taking another sip of coffee, I then left the rest in the car. Getting to the elevator was a hard process. I sometimes have to park across the street. I'd cross the street and finagle my way through broken pieces of side walk, hop up the handicap ramp where the rubber grippers were gone. Relying only on my one leg muscles to get me in. I was proud of myself.

"Hello Sharon, how are you today?"

"The best I can be I suppose. I was wondering if the doctor could put some kind of numbing gel on my wound before she starts debriding? I was also wondering, can I have a blanket, I'm freezing in here. When she looked down at my fingers, they were blue. She stopped what she was doing and got me two warm blankets. Looking to my left were all the familiar tools the doctor used yesterday.

"Here you go my dear."

"I even got it heated for you."

"Oh my God thank you so much. This feels so wonderful."

"Good deal. I wouldn't want you to suffer. I asked the doctor if we could put Lidocaine to numb the wound, and she said yes. After I get the measurements I'll put that on for you."

The warm blankets felt so comforting. Knowing in a few minutes the doctor was going to come in and start tearing my skin off one piece at a time. I was starting to become anxious. I turned my attention to the same pretty blue sea shell curtain for distraction.

"Good morning. I think the cream has sat on long enough so we are going to get started."

I proceeded to hold my foot for her benefit and mine once she grabbed the tweezers. She went back to the same location she'd been working on yesterday."

"I'm sorry. I don't mean to hurt you. Isn't that cream working?"

"Yes, somewhat. That was just a big piece of skin. It seems the little pieces don't hurt as much. Doctor, how long does it usually take a wound like mine to heal?"

"Well that does vary. It's crucial we remove the dead skin so the new pink skin will start growing back. As far as how long, I'd say three to four months if everything goes well."

"Three to four months, that's a long time."

"I've seen worse. Some of my diabetic patients wounds don't heal and they have to have a second amputation. You'll be just fine. Its only your second day and your taking it like a champ."

I thought about what she said as I held my foot with both hands, resting my head on my knees. I drifted away to the ocean playing in the deep blue sea. If it weren't for this peaceful dividing curtain I'd probably loose my mind.

"Your foot feels cold. I'd give you another blanket but we are done for the day. If you look down to the left, you can see we made some good progress. It seems like the numbing cream helped so we will continue using that. Do you have any questions?"

"No Ma'am"

"Okay then. I'll see you tomorrow."

"Alright Sharon. Let me clean that foot and get you out of here."

The nurse grabbed the spray bottle of saline to wash away any bacteria. Then some healing gel and covered the wound with gauze. She got out more gauze and wrapped my foot a little above the ankle. It always felt so much better after it was cleaned and wrapped.

"Nurse, is it normal not sleeping well with this kind of wound? Because I'm having great difficulties, along with phantom pains."

"Yes, it's very common. Especially the phantom pain. It's all neurological. The nerves were separated when they removed your foot and the brain does not acknowledge that your toes are gone. As far as sleep goes, it's going to be very difficult for a while. You will probably get your days mixed with your nights. To find a comfortable position that doesn't hurt or aggravate the nerves it will be a challenge. But it can be done honey. Just hold on to Jesus."

"Yes. Amen to that."

"Ms. Sharon, you are good to go. I didn't wrap it too tight did I?

"No, it's perfect. Thank you for asking the doctor about the cream. I think it helped a lot.

"You're welcome and I agree. It looked less painful. I'm glad I could help with that. Anything that might make you comfortable let us know. That's what we're here for. You have a good day Ms. Sharon."

Feeling thirsty, I bought a sweet tea. Deciding to go sit by the water and drink my tea, I told Jesus I'd see him to tomorrow. Talking to him was the beginning and end of my daily routine. Five days in wound care and two days at home. Either way, I was talking to Jesus.

There wasn't anyone who stepped up to help me. I had to make my own dinner on one foot. Clean house, grocery shop, and comfort myself. Now, I had to learn how to get comfortable with dressing and cleaning my own wound.

Pulling into the parking lot, I rolled down the windows and continued to think about the future. I couldn't see very far. I tried to take it one day at a time or it became overwhelming.

I was really enjoying the smell of the salt water and listening to the waves peaceful rhythm. I closed my eyes, I took a breath and drifted off to the sound of seagulls.

Chapter Fourteen

I wasn't at all comfortable looking at my wound. Cleaning it was difficult too. The black dead skin covered the majority of the wound and that made me nauseous. I thought to myself while making a peanut butter and jelly sandwich for dinner, "it's going to be a long three months of care."

Standing at the kitchen counter eating and drinking my milk, repetitive thoughts wandered. "Who am I now, and what will I do with this amputation and disability." Out loud I spoke in frustration...who will I be Lord? What should I do? I lost my purpose it seemed. I hung my head down, distraught. I saw no end to this horrifying situation.

Until, I heard a soft gentle voice with the answer.

"You will be a writer of books"

For a minute I doubted what I heard. I shrugged my shoulders, ignored it and said, "Sure Lord. I'll be a writer of books."

In severe pain I hopped to my comfortable chair in the living room to watch the evening news and late night shows. Afterwards, I talked my self into getting up to brush my teeth. It was difficult at times to motivate myself. But, It was a long day and I was worn out. Leaning my crutches against the wall close to the bed.

I started thinking about the nurse who was so kind to me today. I thanked God for her. I thanked God for the ability to be independent on one foot and I asked for confirmation "Lord, did you say I'm going to write books?" I heard no answer in return.

So, I laid down in a diagonal position with my feet hanging off the bed. I closed my eyes and drifted off to sleep.

Later, I heard my dog whining. I felt around in the darkness for my crutches."Hey girl. You have to go out?" Hopping to the backdoor I let her out. My foot was on fire and no matter what I did to ease the pain it didn't work. I rubbed it, rocked it, cradled it, prayed on it and still no relief. I was wide awake now, there was no more going back to sleep. This was one of many times I used medical marijuana for the severe pain. It felt like I was walking on hot coals with a pocket knife jabbed in the center and turned with each step. All the while my toes, phantom pains began cramping and there was absolutely nothing I could do to ease the pain of my toes that was surgically removed.

Tears of pain and frustration took over as I slumped my head into my hands. After about twenty minutes the plant began to take away the nerves burning and the cramping stopped. I could now breath! Thanking God for getting me through that rough patch.

I got up, let the dog inside and sat at my dining room table with my laptop. Going directly to make a file called "Books" I began to type with out effort or even a plan. For me, this was a miracle. At this point in time I had two good fingers to type, or rather to peck out the words. But, peck I did. I stayed up from three in the morning until it was time for my wound appointment at eight in the morning. I printed out what I had written, and took it to wound care to help distract me form the excruciating pain I was preparing for.

I made it safely even though I was exhausted. Signing myself in I sat down in the lobby and open what I had written, three chapters. This thing I wrote didn't have a name but as I began to read it, I realized that this was a collection of true short stories of Jesus and I.

It was obvious to me I was to share these supernatural events of the spirit with others. I can tell you I was completely blown away!

Not only did I write this manuscript but it was supernaturally written through me. Wow! Mind Blowing! I thought.

"Miss Bence. Follow me please." the nurse said as she smiled.
I hopped on the table still mesmerized how the Holy Spirit actually told me, I would be a writer of books. Lost in thought the nurse repeated her question.

"Miss Bence. How have you been doing with the wound cleaning?"

"I think pretty good but, it does make me sick to my stomach to see it. Yesterday when I wrapped it back up I held my foot in my hands for the first time."

"That's a good first step. Making peace with your body. How have you been sleeping?"

"Sleep, whats that? I don't sleep well. I get a fire and stabbing feeling that if I happen to fall asleep wakes me instantly."

"I'm sorry. I'm sure it will get better as your wound heals."
This did not give me much hope but it was nice of her to try. She had all the sterile tools out for the doctor. Unfortunately her favorite was the big pointy tweezers.

"Hi Sharon. Sorry I'm late the other patient took longer than anticipated."
Picking up her tweezers I turned my head not to watch.

"Ouch! Damn that hurt!" Jerking my leg away.

"I'm sorry but that was a nice long strip of skin and you'll be glad to know that under it is pretty pink flesh. That's what we need your whole wound to look like." She went back tearing off dead skin while tears began to slowly slide down my cheek after each deliberate tug.

Chapter Fifteen

Six Months Later

Continuously working on my book, it was almost complete. The title picked it's self, Twisted Testimonials. I published it too! You can purchase all the books I've written on Amazon.

How amazing is Jesus. Miracles were being performed daily and I was seeing them. Shoot, I was a part of them! But, unfortunately not my foot. It wasn't healing. I knew it would, but it would be in Gods timing. That, I was firm. I believed this with all my heart. After all of that pain and torture of debridment, my foot was only partially pink with little to no new skin growth after almost a year on crutches. The odds didn't look good.

"Sharon, I'm afraid I'm not getting as far as I hoped with debridment. I believe due to your poor circulation the pink new skin isn't coming in quick enough. So, I think I'm going to move you to the next alternative, the hyperbaric chambers. What this therapy does is increase oxygen to your wound to promote healing quicker. I called your insurance and they will cover twelve weeks. I've scheduled you for today and three times a week. After that treatment I will re evaluate your wound. Hows that sound?"

"So no more yanking off my skin? Ya, I'm game. I'll try anything to get this healed."

I sure was thankful I could take a break from debriding. I was literally about to lose my mind. I really couldn't take it anymore physically or mentally. It was pure torture.

Six months with constant severe pain and nausea. Hopping around like a bunny all the time. I was losing muscle tone in my calf and it was starting to look smaller then the other. My arms were getting really tired and starting to hurt. My hands constantly gripping made my skin tight and painful. Underneath my armpits were tore up from being on the crutches for so long. My shoulder blades were out of wack. I was a mess! How did I handle this extreme change you ask? Jesus.

Hopping to office twenty seven, I opened the door. Standing there my eyes scanned the entire room. There were two glass chambers.

The lights were semi dim. I seen the fire extinguisher, computers, and there were tiny televisions in each chamber.

"Hi I'm Dale, I'll be the nurse that will be motoring you once you get into the chamber. Now, when you get in you're gonna feel like you are going deep underwater. Your ears might pop. There is a television in there to watch or some people go to sleep. The main thing, try to focus on being comfortable and not anxious. I also need you to sign this paper saying that I informed you of what happens in case of an emergency. I would have to depressurize and then follow medical procedure. Do you have any questions?

Stunned, "Um, how long does it take to come up and how long do I have to stay in there?"

"You'll be in there one hour and it takes about ten seconds to decompress the chamber." He gave me a pen to sign the paperwork and showed me where to change into a hospital gown.

"Are you ready?"

"Ready as I'll ever be I guess."
Stepping into the glass chamber was like a space capsule. Extremely small and only room enough to lay on your back. It had a sterile pillow and a blanket inside for comfort. It reminded me of a coffin.

He could hear me and I could hear him through the buzzer system.

"What shows do you like to watch in the morning." I told him as I settled in.

"How is the volume? If it's good we will start to compress. I'll be watching you, so give me a thumbs up once in a while so I know you're doing okay."

I shook my head okay, closed my eyes, took a deep breath and centered. I'm normally not a fearful person. But, I can see how one could have a panic attack in one of these chambers. My ears started popping as if I were flying. I held my nostrils together and blew so I could pop my ears and hear.

That day I was really tired. I closed my eyes. I could tell I was decompressed all the way now. Sensing his eyes on me, I opened mine. Thumbs up he gave me. Thumbs up I returned and then I fell asleep.

"Sharon, it's time to wake up. We're done with therapy. Did you have a restful sleep?"

"I sure did and it was well needed."

"You did real good today."

Waving good bye, I grabbed my crutches and hopped into the elevator, then to my car where I threw the crutches in the backseat.

I sat there for a while resting. The forecast proved to be a hot July summer. Headed for home I seen the statue of Jesus on my way, like everyday. But this day was different.

I felt like an energy pulled into the parking lot. I parked, got out of the car and stood in front of the statue. It was a beautiful bronze carving of Jesus that stood the test of time. Salt from the sea had rusted the base but such intricate work this artist projected.

"Jesus, I am tired. I'm sore." Suddenly, I felt like I was hugged and I desperately needed that. I thanked him for the new therapy and for knowing when I was at my limit. I thanked him for my healing me because I believed in all my heart he died on the cross for our salvation and healing.

Chapter Sixteen

It was the beginning of the week and my calendar was set. Mondays, Wednesdays and Friday were my appointments for the hyperbaric chamber. This week was my fourth week already. It seemed to be going much faster than the debriding. On the opposite days I rested, watched television and got on my I pad. Grocery shopping was on Thursday afternoon. It wasn't an exciting life. In fact it was a life I was struggling with on a daily basis. It was extremely trying emotionally and physically knowing there is no relief for calcinosiss.

"Good morning Sharon. How was your weekend?" Not very interesting, I thought as I gave a wave, walking over to the restroom to change. As I walked out I noticed the other chamber was occupied.

"I see you have another client under."

"Ya, he's about half way though his treatment."
Grabbing the blood pressure cuff he took my blood pressure.

"Okay, hop in, you know what to do."

By this time he knew the programs I liked to watch on television and the volume I preferred. Everything usually ran as clock work. We usually just said a few words to one another and I hopped in the chamber. My visits had become routine.

Turning to stretch my neck, a commercial about laundry detergent came on. As I glanced at the other patient, I became horrified! Instantly I looked for the nurse through the glass chamber, I could see him by the chalk board.

This man is having a seizure and there is nothing I do. Pressing the buzzer, the nurse could heard me. "Help!"
There he is, thank God he heard me. He came running over when I pointed to the patient.

"Mr. Groves can you hear me? The nurse started to bring him up from decompression but it wasn't fast enough. In fact every second felt like a minute too long. Finally, he was up!

"Thank God!"
I watched as his wife come into the room. I couldn't hear what was being said, I just tried to center myself. I could see she was very

worried by the look on her face. Mr. Groves was slumped over to his wheel chair leaning to the right with his eyes closed.

That man could have died in there, my mind raced. Shoot, I could die in here! I made myself get a grip by refocusing my mind. I said a prayer for for him and for myself as I focused my eyes and mind back to my television show I was once enjoying. I took a deep breath.

"Ms. Bence are you okay?"
I gave him a thumbs up. I really didn't want to discuss the situation. It threw me back to my teenage years, when I suffered from epilepsy. Glancing at the clock, fifteen more minutes and I can get out of here. "Hurry Up time." I mumbled.

Chapter Seventeen

Getting into the elevator I thought about the day and how life can end so quickly at any given moment. "It really is precious." The beauty of the way the sun was shining on the water reiterated how life is so beautiful, it made the bay glisten.

I decided to turn right instead of left. "A new direction a new path." I found myself standing on the beach. I closed my eyes just for a minute preparing my balance in the sand. I took a leap of faith. Releasing my wounded foot to meet the other, I stood on both of my feet and allow the good energy from the sea into my soul. How beautiful the water is. It was a place of serenity for me.

Watching the water for possible dolphins to pass by, I scanned the water diligently. Down a couple miles a little boy was fishing with his dad. It reminded me of good memories and put a smile on my face.

So, when you feel like you're in this fight alone and it will never work...trust your faith. You see, this is another one of those times when you can't count on yourself or any other human. For me, I trust Jesus.

Chapter Eighteen

Reaching over to turn off the alarm, I grabbed my crutches and headed for the kitchen. I didn't sleep very well last night and my mouth was dry. Drinking my water I thought, "I wonder if I'll ever have routine sleep or life again." For right now, it was hit and miss. The pain this morning was a seven. I took my medication and unwrapped my wound before I showered.

It was difficult trying to get a good look at it. I tried to take a picture and look at it. I tried to look at it in the mirror. Luckily I was somewhat flexible and could bring my foot to my eyes. This morning it still looked black in the center and only about twenty percent new skin growth. I was concerned. Time had flown by quickly and I knew that this was my last hyperbaric treatment. My wound did not look much better. Cleaning and wrapping it back up I got dressed to head to my appointment.

I never was much of a morning person. When I have a hard time sleeping, its hard for me to focus. Although, it was a beautiful day already. The birds were all out especially the cranes, spoon bills and seagulls. Sailboats were slowly bouncing in rhythm to the waves. The water looked like the night sky with stars scattered and twinkling.

Driving over the bridge my turn off was to the left. "Hi Jesus. Good morning." Passing the statue, I circled for a parking space. There was no handicap parking open or any other spots. Circling the parking lot a few more times a gentleman finally came out and got in his car.

Grabbing my crutches I exited and locked the car. Slipping the crutches under my arms I noticed that my shoulder blades were sore and felt out of place. I really did not have the strength to hop to the door from so far away but I took a deep breath and went along my way.

Crossing the street and hopping up the wheel chair ramp I waited for an elevator. Flexing my foot and leg while I waited I realized that my right leg had become noticeably thinner than my left.

Noticing he was busy chatting with his coworker, I went in the restroom to change my clothes. Once I came out he was ready.

"So how are we doing this fine morning? I bet you're excited about this being your last treatment?"

"I'm tired, didn't get much sleep. Tossing and turning to find a comfortable place on the bed that won't hurt my foot is bothersome. As far as happy the treatment is ending, um, no. I mean I just had high hopes this would heal my wound and I'm afraid it didn't do much. I'm disappointed."

"Ya, I can understand that. I think for those patients like yourself with limited blood flow to the wound it makes it difficult.

"Whats a rough percentage of patients that this therapy heals?'

"I'd say about seventy percent. Those with diabetes have a difficult time with healing. By the way, the doctor wants to check your progress after this appointment."

I nodded my head and then crawled into the chamber. This particular time the television was off and I preferred it that way... Maybe I could catch up on some sleep.

"Sharon, we are through with therapy."

I opened my eyes and looked at him.

"Boy, you had a good nap. Do you feel refreshed?" He asked as he helped me out of the chamber.

"Yes, I do." I went and changed into my clothes. When I came out the nurse shook my hand and wished me luck.

Making my way to see the doctor down the hall I signed in and waited for my name to be called. Looking around the waiting room it was full.

My name was called and I was led to a room.

"How are you Sharon? It looks like you just finished your last hyperbaric treatment today. How did you think it went?" She asked as she gently unwrapped my wound.

"Personally, I think it helped a little bit but not much" There is still a lot of dead skin and the pain is extreme." She looked at my chart then the doctor walked in.

"Hi Sharon let me take a look at that foot of yours. Okay, I can see that I'm going to set you up with an appointment with your orthopedic surgeon. I'd like to have his opinion on why it's taking so long to heal. The receptionist will make your appointment up front when you leave. Do you have questions at this point?"

"Yes, many. So are you telling me my wound won't heal and you're not sure why? That does not leave me with much confidence. Why am I seeing the surgeon again? Where does this leave me. What is the next step?"

"Okay, you're seeing the surgeon to see if he thinks it can heal with the current blood flow to your foot. Your vein test shows that two out of three veins are semi closed and even though they were, that doctor thought you would do fine. As far as the next step I have one more option but, that depends on what the surgeon says. He might think we need to amputate up to the knee where the blood flow is stronger. I know it's easier said than done But, try not to worry. We will get you healed one way or another. Oh, by the way, your doing a great job keeping the wound clean. Truly I'm surprised it hasn't gotten infected after all this time being open."

I was dumbfounded. It was like I heard what she said but didn't comprehend it. As the nurse came in to wrap my foot for the two hundredth time my face had a flat effect. I was in shock, I was!

I didn't know what I expected her to say but, I didn't expect her to say I might need another amputation. The whole day was a blur after that appointment. I went home and went to sleep.

Chapter Nineteen

Upon my arrival I checked in at the front desk and helped myself to some coffee. Sitting down, I looked around the room. There were many patients with missing limbs.

Still on crutches, after nine months, my arms and back were becoming an issue. I seen a gentleman about six feet tall wearing a veterans hat. I smiled at him, as we made eye contact and asked him how he was.

He answered and told me about his injury. A mine exploded while he was in a field. He had his left leg amputated up to his hip. He was kind and had a great sense of humor. I explained my condition. Soon thereafter I was called back to see the orthopedic surgeon.

"So, how are we doing today?" I nodded my head. I didn't want to hear what he had to say really. I had full confidence that my God would indeed heal me on his time.

"It looks like we need to schedule another surgery to amputate up to your knee. Its been nine months and by reading the report from your wound doctor, everything she's tried hasn't worked. I truly believe it's due to the lack of circulation and with out good blood flow to the wound, it won't heal."

I began to tear up. Afraid he would say exactly that. I took a deep breath. "Doctor, I understand you're coming from a medical perception. But, I trust Jesus has me healed me. It's not infected, so why the rush to chop off my calf?"

"Well that's just it, it's been open almost a year and you and your God are getting no where. I'll have the nurse schedule a date for surgery."

"Wait one second, I don't agree to surgery. My faith tells me it will heal, maybe not on your time but, on God's time." I was appalled at his response and beginning to become more upset with him. We were trying out talk to one another civilly. But, both of our voices became stern and a little louder.

"Well, that's the first time I've heard that. I understand what you hope will happen but religion has it's place and I'm telling you it has no chance to heal." He became frustrated with me. I believed that My God died on the cross so that I could be healed with all my heart.

"If we can't agree then there is no need for further discussion." He walked out of the room in anger and slammed the door. I sat there in tears feeling raked over the coals by his words and tone. I then wiped my tears, held my head high and proceeded to the nurses station to check out.

"Are you okay dear?"

"Yes I'm just upset. The doctor was rude how he addressed my situation. I grabbed a root beer sucker to calm me down.

"I am so sorry. He is head strong like that."

"Well, he told me not to come back so I won't. You've been great though and I appreciate it so much. Bye now."

My head was in a whirlwind. I didn't know what to do and neither did any of the doctors. In fact my wound doctor remark was, "Most of my patients are older diabetics and and usually pass away if the wound doesn't heal. You on the other hand I have no idea what to do with."

When I got out of the elevator I asked God for his guidance. I said "The doctors don't know how to heal me Lord. What should I do?" Sobbing in the car my mind was churning trying to think of a possible fix. I put the car in gear to headed home. At the stop sign, still sniffling, I heard God!

Right now you're probably thinking either,

oh ya sure you did, or you're praising God with me. I've herd him talk to me before so I knew it was him. He's usually very direct and this was no different.

"Call Dr. Hernandez."

"What Lord? You want me to call a doctor?" I reiterated. I herd no reply.

Instantly, I got out a pen to write the name down so I wouldn't forget. I thanked him profusely. When I returned home I looked up the name on the internet. You would think there would be more than one doctor with that name. But, no. Low and behold there he was!
Dr. Hernandez!

I was in shock and awe. Completely amazed and so very grateful for God's guidance. Dialing the number with great excitement, I made an appointment. Coincidentally, he was in the same hospital my wound doctor was in. I was so excited, and at ecstatic, I knew my faith would get me through, if only I counted on my God, and he did.

After I hung up the phone I did a little jitterbug dance, throwing my crutches and caution to the wind. Praising God for all his goodness and his direction. Then, I suddenly realized, this was the very first time I stood on my own without crutches. I waited to fall... But, I didn't. So, I continued to dance and sing "Thank you Jesus, for your guidance. Dear

Jesus, I love you." Giving it a tune, snapping my fingers, I kept repeating it with such joy and enlightenment it began to fill my heart.
I could feel a miracle was on it's way!

Chapter Twenty

Waking up that morning, I had energy like I never knew I had!
I made myself breakfast, washed the dishes and mopped the floor while singing. It seemed for the first time in a long time I felt human and not just handicapped.

I witnessed a miracle yesterday! That lightened my load one hundred tons. I walked around in bliss! Overcome with the Lords direction. Dreaming of what will come next. I could finally see the light at the end of the tunnel.

You see, I've learned many important lessons during this monstrous ordeal. First, the only one you can truly depend on is your higher power. People may love you but, sometimes they can't be there for you. It could be geographic location, emotionally unavailable or unawareness. It could also be that this difficult time was meant for you to grow stronger in body, mind and spirit. To get to know God.

Personally, by turning to him with my troubles, I know he's listening and I know his promises. This gets me through life.

The next thing I learned was not to believe what you see or hear. But, to believe in what you know in your heart to be true. Do not succumb to the disease. Meaning, the fight over the mind over matter as just begun.

I knew I would be healed. Shoot, I never accepted this disease from day one. I treated the symptoms and thanked God for healing me everyday. I truly have many scars from the calcinosis and I type with my two middle fingers because the others are disformed or amputated.

However, I don't see my hands in this way. I simply don't judge them. I see them functional and healed even though it has it's daily challenges. Like when I travel out of the country the supervisor always needs to be called over to verify that it is me and theses are my hands. Why you ask? I have no fingerprints. The ulcers took them away. It's interesting how children are very perceptive. They seem to notice my scars and missing parts with empathy, compassion and curiosity. I just tell them I have a boo-boo or ouchy, its a universal word that all children know. They definitely understand.

Adults hardly notice unless I have visible scars or ulcers on my face. With this diagnosis you can't be vain or play the martyr. You must disown this disease or any type of sickness. Deny it, and thank God for his help.

You might say my life is a success story. A patient with Scleroderma, thriving after thirty years with perfect blood counts, perfect organ functions and a positive attitude. Is that why I'm still around with this disease? You might ask, Is she filled with so much hope that she literally walks in peace and hope? Seeing her life with a new outlook, a different view or perspective?

"Yes. I tell you." It was something that never wavered in my mind. I was going to fight! I was going to be strong in my faith. I was going to believe in supernatural blessings and promises. The outcome was just as mind blowing to me as it is to you.

Chapter Twenty One

Today was the big day! What would the doctor say I wondered.
I looked around the room and smiled at an older lady that had her foot in a brace. Then I was called back. The nurse took my vitals and entered the information. Then she left.
Looking out the window at the beautiful body of water where the the sail boats glided slowly across the bay. The sun rays danced in visible sight. I became lost in thought when I heard the door open. I was startled at my name being called.
"Sharon, where have you been? I've been waiting for you?" He asked with such wonder.
My eyes got so big! The hair on my arms and neck stood straight up! I had no way to answer to his question. I was dumbfounded.

How could I even articulate the answer to such a supernatural question? This was God!

Snapping out of my shock, I turned my attention to what the doctor was saying.

"I think what I need is do is remove skin from your hip. Debride what the wound doctor couldn't. After that, I'll transfer the healthy skin from your thigh to your amputation. In theory it will attach its self and grow healthy skin over your wound" He then smiled.

"Wow that sounds pretty simple to me and quite ingenious!" I smiled too.

"Great, sounds like we have a plan! On your way out schedule a surgery date with the receptionist. He then stunned me with his words.

"I'm glad we finally met."

Still in revelation over his words and the quick fix to heal my foot, I was in amazement! I made my appointment and decided to go directly over to see the sailboats.

Sitting there with a heart filled with peace and serenity. I was completely overcome by the grace of God. It was one year on this very date that I had my foot amputated. Was it a coincidence that on this day God sends me to the doctor of his choosing? I started daydreaming about getting rid of the crutches and envisioned myself walking and dancing with balance and grace. I have to admit, with or without my foot, I was happier than id ever been.

I was so inspired once home, that I typed several chapters on my first book, Twisted Testimonials. My goal was to get my foot healed and complete my first book so I could get it on the market.

Chapter Twenty Two

Today was the day I'd been waiting for. Checking myself in for outpatient surgery, I complemented a lady on her skirt and sat down. Waiting for my angel to open the door, I stared out the window of floating sailboats, he called my name.

"Are you ready for surgery Sharon?" Shaking my head with a big smile he knew he didn't need to hear my words to understand my excitement.

"Great, I will have the nurse show you to the prep room."

The surgical technicians wheeled me down with my gown on and the warm blankets I requested. I was so ready to take this giant step! I closed my eyes until they reached the operating room. Thinking, today was the first step in healing my wound I thought. Then everything went dark.

Returning to the recovery room I was extremely groggy. I couldn't remember what happened or where I was. All I knew, was I had the best sleep Id ever had in my life. As I slowly woke up the nurse dismissed me with instructions and my daughter drove me home. She left, and I took a nap. By the time I woke up it was nine in the evening, it was time for bed.

I couldn't help but think that soon all of this suffering would be coming to an end. The doctor that Jesus recommended was the best!

Grabbing my crutches that were leaning against the beige textured wall, a thought popped into my mind. "I am so very ready to finally get rid of these crutches! I wonder if I'll be able to walk or if I'll need special shoes? Would I need a cane or crutches for stability?" I had a lot of questions running around in my mind.

With nothing good to watch on television, and I just had eaten dinner, I decided to start working on my book.

Chapter Twenty Three

Truthfully, I starting to get my days confused. I wasn't on a routine like I was when I was working. Then, I scheduled for sleep. Now I took slept when I could. The pain was bothering me on my foot and forearm continually. I'd eat when I was hungry and watch a little television. If I couldn't sleep, I'd get up to work on my book. I had a goal to finish them both by the end of the year, and that was one thing I was was good at, being goal oriented.

It was the weekend, time to clean the house. Instead of picking up the laundry with both hands, I would kick the pile with my working foot or use my crutches. For bathing, I was still covering the dressing with a plastic bag so my wound didn't get wet. When I mopped I stood on one foot and hopped. When I got tired I would sit and reach as far as I could.

Thinking about all the possibilities of walking again was getting exciting. Next Friday would be one week since he took the skin from my thigh and grafted it on to my open wound.

Until now, I had put no significant weight on my amputated foot. Slowly I started on it each day. Prepping my mind and foot for a new beginning and an end to this exhausting trauma.

Chapter Twenty Four

The days went by quickly and it was finally Friday. I woke up in the best mood. I didn't have to wait long at the office which was a blessing. Sitting on the table, staring out the window seeing the sailboats, made me feel calm.

The door opened "Well how's my favorite patient?"

"If I heard those three magical words. You are healed. I'd be on top of the world!"

He gloved up and unwrapped my foot. It always felt cold and naked when it was unwrapped. I watched as he took out the gauze in my heel. "That looks pretty good to me." He then checked the prognosis of the graft and unwrapped my forearm.

"Well in my eyes, everything is looking good. Your wound on your heel and arm healed well and your graft is taking to the skin. I think you're on your way to healing. I'd probably give it one more month or so. Then I can truly say those words you so desperately want to hear. If you have some time today, I want you to get fitted for a special pair of shoes with a kick plate."

"What's a kick plate and why will I need special shoes?

"Since your toes are gone, the foot needs something to push off your step to walk. Without having toes you'll find that you will not have the balance you once did. Make an appointment for next month on your way out."

I didn't care if my toes were gone. I was too excited to go see what shoes I could pick out. For me, shoes were my obsession! I loved wearing heels to work and diversifying my look with the right shoe and handbag.

I pulled up to the orthopedic shoe store and checked in. They asked me to fill out some forms. After I did, I returned them and sat back down. Thumbing through the magazine he called my name, I followed him into a room with about ten pairs of shoes.

"Are these the only choices you have to choose from?"

"Yes." He answered while measuring my foot then putting foam in the shoe. After that he took an impression of my foot and put a piece metal in to give me the kick back they said I needed.

"Wait a minute! I have to pay ninety dollars for a shoe that I don't even like? I could put a sock where you put the toe filler in. I really don't think I need a kick plate. I think I'm gonna go with another alternative." A little perturbed that there were no shoes to my liking.

"Okay Ma'am. If you change your mind just give us a call and we'll get you on the schedule. Thank you for coming. You have a nice day."

I thanked him, got in the car and headed home to try on the shoes in my closet.

Still with a smile and hope in my heart, I went in my bedroom closet and began pulling every pair of shoes out. The heels were a no go. There was no way I could stand at an angle with no toes. I set them all in a bag. Next, I tried on my flats. I found that the cut in all my flats were too high and my foot would fall right out. They went in the bag as well.

My tennis shoes seemed to work well. I stuck two or three socks in the toe area, tried them on, and tied them up.

The end of my foot hit where the end of the tongue was on the shoe. It was a light weight shoe and seemed to work so I put them both on. Unbelievably I took my first step with my crutches for support. It felt weird finally wearing a shoe but I knew I could use this method instead of paying ninety dollars for shoes.

The next group I tried on, were my boots. The ones with a heel was a no go, but the ones that were flat I could wear. The last group were my Crocs. These I could wear as well. It made me a little sad, when I realized that I would never be able to walk into a shoe store and pick out a pair of shoes.

Taking the bag, I loaded it up in my car to give to the Salvation Army. Even though I was aware I'd never work again, I kept my dresses and work suits. I guess maybe in the back of my mind I thought maybe I would go back to work or need them for some reason.

I was still uncomfortable not having a job and no schedule. Yet a writer writes whenever a writer has time to write. So, I focused on that goal to take my mind off of my amputation.

Within that month before I seen Dr. Hernandez, I worked diligently. My only goal was to focus on publishing my second book titled, "Thought I Knew The Plan." The first book, "Twisted Testimonials." I wrote quickly and it was published.

Though there were consequences from typing so long with only two fingers. They became stiff and extremely sensitive. It was hard to pick up objects such as my coffee cup, and at any given moment I had the burden of accidentally hitting them wrong or dropping the object.

Chapter Twenty Five

At this particular time in my life I had calcinosis on my knees, ears, cuticles, fingers, tailbone, chin and forehead. After thirty years of living with this disease, I never claimed it in my heart.

I made sure I took care of myself mentally, emotionally, spiritually and physically.

The hard part of treating Scleroderma, CREST SYNDROME, is that there isn't much funding for research due to its rarity. Most specialist and those studying Scleroderma don't have any break through regarding calcinosis. (8/2019)

I spoke with two great specialist a few months back in Houston Texas. Both were top notch when it came to knowing the newest

treatments of the disease. One of them was from Texas and worked in research and studies of Scleroderma. The other Doctor flew from Italy. He was also one of the top doctors in his country regarding
Scleroderma.

I had one question for them both. Is there any new treatment that can reduce or delete the growth and relieve the excruciating pain from calcinosis?

Their answer was "NO." As far as how to stop or treat the growth of calcinosis. There was also no effective way to treat the high pain level that runs with the diagnosis of Scleroderma. They did however, have some breakthrough regarding pulmonary issues.

Chapter Twenty Six

What Does CREST Stand for?

(C) Calcinosis~ For me the most difficult to deal with is the Calcinosis and ulcers. My Doctor prescribed Tramodol for pain.
It doesn't take the pain away, it just brings my pain down a level. So again, I use Gods plant. This brings my pain level down to a one where I can function through the day without severe pain.

(R)Reynauds~ I currently take Sidenifil for my circulation. It took my doctor some time to get the insurance to pay for this. It's generic Viagra and works very well for me.

(E) Esophageal~ Dysfunction such as acid reflux (Gerd).

My doctor has me on Nexium. I have noticed throughout the years
my body can become immune to the medications, so we switch. My
swallowing is delayed and was diagnosed with Barrett Disease.

(S) Sclerodactyly~ Is the thickening of skin mainly on my fingers
and face.

(T) Telanglectasis~ The tiny red busted blood vessels. They are all
over my body. More so on my face, hands and chest. Doctors don't
seem concerned about them much. I hardly give dilation of
capillaries a second thought.

I've also suffered from low Iron. They found that I was bleeding internally with a colonoscopy test. However, it was easily fixed. The doctor just cauterized the wound shut.
The key to it all... not to let yourself get overwhelmed. No worries! That can go for anything. The kids, animals, work, disease, lack of sleep, all stress. Find a way to keep yourself in balance, and in peace.
Remember, you woke up today and that

alone is a blessing. "Why should you be grateful?" You probably wonder.

I understand. I know where you are. It is so important to be grateful and thankful because It out wits the disease. Mind over matter is of utmost importance.

Upon further examination and personal experience I conclude that stress will make your disease worse too. It can even be the main cause of death. Make sure of one thing, you value a peaceful mind and heart. This will buy you many years of a happiness.

Chapter Twenty Seven

Today was my appointment with Dr. Hernandez. It had been a month since I saw him last. I had been working very hard on balance and on my walking without support of the crutches. I was starting to accept what my foot could do instead of what It couldn't. I'm now comfortable with putting pressure on it and familiar with my foot again. In my mind it was always healed, and those were the words I so desperately wanted the doctor to confirm.

Waiting, looking out of the window at the bay and the sailboats, hoping this was the last time I would have to come back to this hospital. Thanking Jesus for his healing power.

The door opened and I became startled. Turning around with a smile we greeted one another. Instead of asking me to sit on the examination table he strolled over to where I was sitting. We both sat enjoying the view.

"Such a serene view of the bay."

"Yes, I agree. It's my serenity for sure. I love the water. It will be so great when I can get back to swimming."

"Hold on now, let me take a quick peak before you go jumping in the water already."

Slipping off my Crocs and socks, I showed him my foot. I had my legs crossed as he held my foot in his hand pulling where he stitched the skin in different areas. Smiling he said "Well, I think we've done it. It looks really great!"

"Wonderful can I hear those three sweet words I've been longing to hear for over a year?" Closing my eyes, anxiously I waited to hear the next words he would speak.

"Sharon, you are healed!"
Standing up with tears in my eyes, I asked him to please say it one more time.

He obliged. "Sharon, you are healed."

Grabbing his hand with utter excitement, I asked if we could pray. He said he was a Christian too. We sat by the window in our two comfy chairs holding hands. I thanked God for sending me to him. Thanked him for the doctors steady hand and keen eye. Thanked him for his direction and his unconditional love. We both said Amen. We stood up and I thanked him for his work, for listening to God and for giving me a new life.

"I'll miss you believe it or not." I said with a tear.

"I'm sure you'll be going zero to ten in no time flat." He smiled and gave me a big hug before he walked out of the door.

I just sat for a minute taking all the good news in. After gathering myself I walked in amazement. I walked in grace. My loving Jesus sent me here, and I finally heard those three words I longed to hear for thirteen months.

"Thank you Jesus!" Crying with joy opening the heavy office door. I moved slowly toward the elevator in complete awe. But, to my surprise I couldn't move one step further. Subconsciously I dropped to my knees. My hands folded and my head touching the ground. Sobbing with adoration and appreciation. I yelled out loud...

"I AM HEALED!"

Things That Helped Me

1. Keep your stress low and listen to your body.
2. Vitamin E oil on ulcers. As well as Silver Sulfadiazine were good options. Vitamin K, Primrose, Omega, Gaba and a double dose of multivitamin for Women I take daily.
3. Lidocaine Ointment 5% works for debriding the calcinosis out of the skin.
4. Drink three vitamin shakes daily.
5. Soak in a hot tub. Add natural salts and oils. Jet tub is best.
6. Treat yourself to a hot mineral springs bath. I found one in New Mexico, in the town of Truth and Consequences. Staying in the water took away many deposits of calcinosis. I was truly amazed. If I have calcinosis that is so painful I can't bare, I soak that part in a bowl. It dissolves the calcinosis.
It's well worth the trip and make sure you bring plenty gallon jugs with you to take

home some water with you.
7. Use an electric facial scrubber to help to loosen calcinosis.
8. Medical Marijuana for pain.
9. Get plenty of rest and become proactive when going to the doctor. Chances are you know whats right for you.
10. Cast your cares on your higher power. Refuse to worry. Refuse to accept your diagnosis by saying repetitively, my body is healed. My cells are moving into alignment. Most of all stay positive!

Living with Scleroderma

Living with Scleroderma

Living with Scleroderma

Living with Scleroderma